The Silly Things That Make Us Sick, Fat and Old

Gordon R. Keiser

The Silly Things That Make Us Sick, Fat and Old

The A. I. M. Program

A Breakthrough Health Education Series

Foreword

When I look back at my life a few years ago I see an old man, sick with lots of medicines. I was a diabetic, with high blood pressure, lots of cholesterol, way overweight and a brain on the way out. I was like most of the people my age. I was spending most of my time being inactive, watching TV, reading and planning for my next doctor's visit so I could tell him how much my joints hurt. I really expected sympathy, but instead I got a lecture about the road I was heading down if I didn't change my life.

By this time I was about forty pounds overweight, with a belly that required a belt 10 inches longer than I needed when I had been a young man. My doctor said "Mr. Keiser, you are going to have to take this diabetes seriously or some bad things are going to start happening to you". He continued by saying "you are at very high risk of heart attack, stroke, sight loss and other bad things". When I asked him what I should do he said, "You are going to have to get active and lose weight". I asked him how I could do that. He really did not have the time to get into it but told me that my health care provider did some have some good classes that may help.

It wasn't until later when I started thinking about what it would be like once you had a stroke or heart attack if you lived through it. I hated the thought of being confined to a bed or wheel chair and having to have people take care of me. I loved the thought of living an independent life and going where I wanted to and when I wanted to. Although I was in my sixties I was just not ready to admit I was "old". I had seen plenty of seniors that continued an active and productive life and I wanted to be one of those people.

I signed up for the course on diabetes and looked forward to the day the class started. The class was a number of weeks in length and was held in a class room style. We got lots of information from people who were very well educated with lots of certificates. It was very apparent that these people did not have diabetes and were not going though what we were. We watched movies and slide presentations and carried home a major boat load of paper. I never heard from those people again. It was as if: here take this ton of information and figure out how to implement it in your life.

When I got home I tried to remember what the instructors said in class. I looked thought my written information to try to make sense of the life style changes I was going to have to make to turn things around. Wait... What? I was going to have to make changes in my life style? Oh, no I just want to take something to make it all better. That was where it really started. You find that all of that medicine does nothing to bring about a "cure". The next time you go to your doctor they increase the dosage or add an additional pill.

I wanted to find out what was causing my health problems and what would change it for the better. I didn't want to just take more and more medicine. I started reading everything I could find. I subscribed to newsletters from teaching hospitals, universities, laboratories, and governmental agencies, magazines and newspapers. My files started to fill up and my bank account went the other direction.

Often times I would find a pearl of wisdom that I could actually use in my life. The first real breakthrough was the discovery of the use of journalizing to record my health indicators on a daily basis. The indicators were ones we have all heard of. They were simple to do, could be done in my home without running to a lab every day. I could afford the equipment and they actually reflected what was going on. By writing things down I could see what was helping and what did not have much of an effect. Here is what I started recording every day, first time in the morning: blood pressure, heart rate, blood sugar, steps taken and my belly size. Notice I did not use weight since it is not a good reflection of general health. Journalizing was a real revelation on so many levels. I could see what made a difference and what didn't. I could begin to feel good about myself as things began to improve. I had real numbers to talk about not just subjective feelings. Now I could separate the "nice to know" information coming out of science from the information that had a practical application in my life and its effect.

The next direction my research had taken was to find out what causes poor health. By this time I had changed my career from a fat old retired guy to a health researcher.

Along the way I began to see that much of the scientific research being done is so narrow and specialized that it is hard to apply to our everyday life. But, never the less, I did find situations or things that have a negative effect on our health. Many things by themselves may have little effect but when a host of situations come together they can be really bad.

Many of the things having a bad effect on our health are not the things health care professionals are warning us about. Here is a good example: loss of sleep, poor self concept, worry and disengagement with society. Many health care professionals tell us we need to be more active and get better nutrition.

I found that it is not that simple. Turns out that poor health is a complex of causes many of which we have never heard of,

The first step is to look at what makes us sick and that is chapter one. The second step is to look at the control points that profoundly affect our health and our enjoyment in life and our very relationships with others. Step three is to look at what changes we can make in our style of life to bring about great and good health. Step four looks at what tools are included in the AIM Program to help you make the changes that will benefit your short term and long term health. The fifth chapter identifies the positive and delicious changes that have been proven by scientific research, personal experience and feedback from others involved in the AIM Program.

Be sure to get your "Starter Kit" from our website at: www.activityismedicine.com to get properly started on this wonderful journey. Good luck and be sure to bring someone else along.

Table of Contents

The silly things that make us fat, sick and stupid

When I first started to research the things that were making me and most of the people I know sick, fat and stupid, I expected to find that my problem was what I was eating and my not getting enough exercise. That is simple right? Everybody knows that! But, I had tried dieting and it never worked very long for me. Most of my friends and family were having little success with a whole range of conventional and off the wall approaches. Of course we all lost a few pounds to begin with but then we would all gain it back and most of the time double. It was as if our bodies were telling us who really was in charge. Don't get me wrong, we all know that eating a well balanced diet is good for us, but what does that mean? It took me the longest to figure out the nutrition part of the program.

I had also joined the gym and like most people saw little results. So maybe just dieting or just exercise is not the answer to good health.

I keep reading and found that having a positive outlook helps. I found a scientific study that showed patients with cancer responded better to treatment when they had a positive outlook, watched a lot of comedy, laughed a lot and had a supportive base of people around them. It wasn't until much later I learned why a positive attitude really does help good health.

I then found a research study that talked about toxins and their effect on the immune's systems response. Seems that when the immune system is busy processing toxins there is less of it to go around to keep you safe and healthy. Not only that, but the liver tends to use that highly processed food you are eating (toxin) to make fat and lipids (cholesterol) which helps keep you fat and sick. Toxins are all around us and we can not protect ourselves from all of them. I came to realize that if we do many of the things that improve the immune system we can handle many toxins and still retain or repair our health.

I came upon a scientific study that shows that being inactive gets us into a downward spiral. This one negative item was implicated in more health problems than any other single situation. The other side of that coin showed that adding activity to your day improved more health situations than any other situation. That is when I bought the domain name: activityismedicine.com because it was turning out to be true that activity really was better than most medicine without all the side effects.

The silly things that make us fat, sick and stupid

Laboratories are busy doing scientific research on stress. We have all heard the saying: "stress can kill you". First I had to find out what stress really was. Then I had to come to know what I could do to reduce the effects of stress and include those things into my life. Turns out there are lots of things that cause us stress but stress is self imposed meaning mostly it is something we do to ourselves. If we do it to ourselves how can we change our thoughts and actions to do less of it?

Next was negative outlook. Doctors have for a long time known that people who have a positive outlook and a strong support of people who are positive, respond to cancer treatment better that those who tend to be more negative. Wow, it even improves cancer treatment? But why is that true? Further research in that area allowed me to see the mechanisms involved. As I continued researching health problems and their causes I found a common thread pointing to what I called "control points".

I then found that a lack of positive feedback leads to health problems. As most of us know when we a going to school, raising a family, building a career we are constantly receiving feedback to how we are doing. Most is positive and helps us to continue to improve and receive more positive feedback. It is like an upward spiral. The opposite happens when we retire. For the most part, feedback comes to a screeching halt. The kids are gone, no more job to gain feedback from, little contact with fellow workers, no learning challenges and unless we inject challenges into our life we gain little feedback.

As a senior we have more time to worry. For some reason seniors find the ability to worry about things that will never come true. We seniors seem to be able to make up things to worry about. Worry brings about an increase in cortisol (the stress hormone) and a decrease in dopamine and endorphin (positive life building hormones). This situation starts the downward spiral that unless we make positive life style changes, can lead us into major health problems.

Along with worry we seem to disconnect from our children, our friends and life in general. The loneliness, loss of hope, disengagement and poor self-esteem all leads to the same downward path to poor and increasingly poor health.

Now we are bombarded by "The Biggest Looser" TV program as if exercise is the total answer, yet most of the people gain their weight back within one year of being on the show.

It is funny that if you ask someone "what leads to good health and wellness" it really does depend on who you ask.

A friend of mine gave me a copy of a movie called "Fat, Sick and Almost Dead to watch. It is a story about a guy who travels across American on a liquid fast of fresh fruits, vegetable, nuts and beans in an attempt to get his health back. He finds his health, loses a lot of weight and gains a brand new life style. I don't believe that juicing can work as a long term life style although it is a great way to get back to a healthy body.

A few weeks ago someone sent me a video designed to sell me a colon cleanser. According to the video getting the food to move through your body can solve all your health problems and you will live happily ever after.

When I talk to physical trainers they tend to feel that if you are not healthy you are just not working out hard enough.

I've been told that meditation can have a profound effect on your health. Next, I bought supplements designed to bring you the uppermost health. The list goes on with herbs, straw extract, rohodiola, and on and on.

Turns out there is not "just one thing" that will turn your health around. Yes, exercise is important, yes, nutrition is important, but did you know that self esteem will make you sick? Worry will increase the cotisol level in your blood and then it becomes a toxin which raises havoc with your cells. Then there is a negative outlook, a lack of positive feedback, lose of sleep, stress, loss of hope, non-engagement with society and they all have a negative effect on your health and wellness.

The human body is way, way too complex to think that changing one thing will fix everything. That is like thinking that changing your car's oil will fix that low air pressure in your tire. They are connected: keeping them both in balance will make your car run better and last longer.

In the early years of health research I felt overwhelmed. I wondered, "How could I ever know all I needed to know about a complex system like the human body"? Then someone told me about the science of "control points". It is like operating you car. You do not have to know how a four cycle internal combustion motor works to use it. You only need to know how to start it, how to use the accelerator, the brakes and that little button that makes the window go up and down. Those are the control points.

Turns out there are control points for the body. What I find amazing is that they are not at all what you think they are. They are all hormones. I guess if you are a medical professional these may not be so surprising to you but I find that most people are really surprised. Hormones are crucial substances the body uses to communicate with various systems and are raw materials used by all cells of the body.

At first I thought we were talking about testosterone and estrogen. That's all I thought there was. Turns out there are hundreds of hormones each with its job to do and many have numerous jobs.

I found that of the hundreds of hard working hormones in the body, there is only a handful of hormones that are the control points. Having the proper amount in our systems brings about good health, energy, a positive outlook, self confidence and on and on. Not having the proper balance of some of these hormones allows bacteria and virus to take hold and make us sick, run down, fat, and old before our times.

Here is the list of hormones I found that act as the "Control Points". These are the substances that, when they are available to the body in the right balance, help us recover and stay well or when they are out of proportion, allow sickness, are responsible for weight gain and let some of our cells grow out of control:
- Dopamine
- Endorphin
- Serotonin
- Melatonin
- Insulin Receptors
- Cortisol

Conventional health care stays away from talking about this because there is no way to make money from it. All of these hormones are made in the brain. What? Wait! I thought the brain was for thinking and memory. Well, the brain is also the most fantastic pharmacy in the universe. It manufactures hundreds of hormones on demand, (if you have supplied it with the proper raw materials). Oh, that is why nutrition is so important? Some of the brain manufactured hormones are also made in other areas of the body but the primary source is the brain.

Here however, is a double edged sword! You can't go to the drug store and get your dopamine nor can you get an injection from your doctor. No one has ever been able to make it. Even if they did, it doesn't last very long and you would get addicted to it.

There is a real advantage to have the manufacturing plant between your ears. When you need it, your brain can make it. Too bad there is not a switch for it that you could just press when you needed to feel good. For now you have to rely on thoughts or actions. What? Wait! You can make dopamine by what you do and what you think? Cool! Here are some good examples of actions you can take to stimulate the production of dopamine: pet your cat, watch a sunset, solve a problem, eat a chocolate, have sex or think a pleasant thought.

Ok, let's put this together. The body needs sufficient amounts of dopamine to help build and repair our body's cells. We can stimulate the production of dopamine by thinking a positive thought as well as other thoughts and actions. So we can just sit around and make ourselves healthy. No, remember good health is not "Just". Our thoughts and attitudes do help in the good health game but we also need movement to put it into play.

That is the breakthrough that the A. I. M. Program brings into our everyday life. In doing the research I found that what makes us sick, fat and clouds our brains is our everyday life. Wait! What? Our everyday style of life makes us sick? You bet it does!

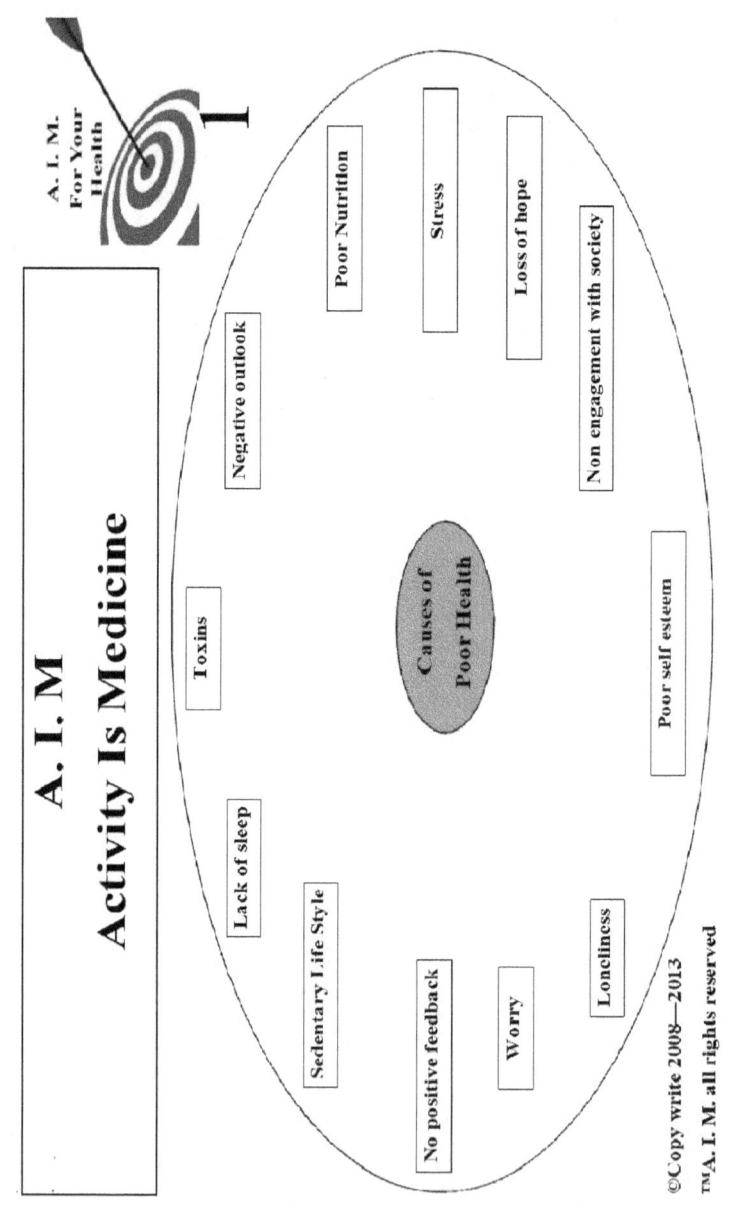

A. I. M
Activity Is Medicine

A. I. M.
For Your
Health

Causes of Poor Health

- Poor Nutrition
- Stress
- Loss of hope
- Non engagement with society
- Poor self esteem
- Loneliness
- Worry
- No positive feedback
- Sedentary Life Style
- Lack of sleep
- Toxins
- Negative outlook

The Control Points that drive our health

Control points are like the parts of the automobile we use to control it, such as a steering wheel, brakes, accelerator and all those dash buttons. We don't have to understand how the internal combustion engine works to use its abilities. We just have to know how to use the control points.

Since it is a known fact the level of certain hormones can cause poor health or help us get and stay healthy. Effecting the production or reductions of those hormones will affect our health even more than our doctor or medicine ever can. We are going to take a look at some of the most toxic and also most life affirming hormone and then see how to effect their production. The ones I have chosen I call The "AIM Control Points". There may be other hormones that could act as control points but, these are well studied and well understand by science. In addition, we know how to effect them.

On the following page you will find a graphic of the control points. I've shown them enclosed in a circle because they do have a lot of interaction and some hormones affect other hormones. As an example let's say you accomplish an import project: the body will produce an increased level of dopamine and endorphin to make you feel happy, confident and a feeling of general euphoria. The hormone melatonin will also increase and you will sleep better.

Cortisol

Of all the Control Point hormones, cortisol is the only one with negative side effects. It starts out as very positive because it is the hormone that helps us get through scary situations. It has been called the "fight or flight" hormone. We can handle high levels of cortisol for short periods of time but within about twenty minutes it turns into a toxin and starts killing cells. It has been called the "primary stress hormone" and in our modern busy life style it is making us lose sleep, gain weight, and suffer a whole list of health problems.

In the distant past the hunt and kill was over quickly and cortisol levels began to recede. In today's lifestyle we worry, have stressful jobs, and find lots of other situations to increase our cortisol level.

Recent research shows that chronically elevated cortisol levels makes us fat, thins our bones, shrinks our brains, suppresses our immune system, saps our energy levels and kills our sex drive. It also elevates our blood sugar, increases our blood pressure, and changes our memory and moods. That is the bad news and it is really, really bad news because it is so ubiquitous. It happens a little at a time so you don't notice it creeping up on you (jobs, kids, traffic, bills and etc).

Cortisol is the stress hormone and the more of it you have, the more stressed you feel...the more vulnerable to disease you are and the faster you age! The Good News is that you can do something about it.

The AIM Program can help. Through an easy to follow program called AIM you can learn how to incorporate stress management, exercise, activity and diet into a very doable approach to daily life. Some of the following chapters will lead you through the "how to" processes of reducing cortisol and some are as easy as meditating or simply listening to the AIM Meditation CD.

Dopamine

Just talking about the Control Point hormone called dopamine gives me a warm and fuzzy feeling. After all, it is the hormone that floods our body when we are petting our cat, watching a beautiful sun set, eating chocolate, a warm shower, having sex or any activity that makes us smile and feel good.

Dopamine is one of the more studied hormones and a lot is known about it and its effect on our bodies and our very health. Dopamine is a key determinant of physiological age and resistance to disease. When levels are low, you're more susceptible to aging and disease; when they're high, the body is at its peak—vibrant, healthy, and able to fight disease successfully.

Endorphins

The Control Point hormone Endorphin always makes me think of dolphins playfully swimming along in clear blue waters. Endorphins resemble the effects of morphine giving us a feeling of well-being. They are produced by the pituitary gland and the hypothalamus during exercise, excitement, pain, consumption of spicy food, love and orgasm. Endorphins are implicated in helping in the repair and production of the bodies' cells.

Serotonin

Serotonin plays an important part in the regulation of learning, mood, sleep and vasoconstriction (constriction of blood vessels). Experts say serotonin also might have a role in anxiety, migraine, vomiting and appetite.

Alterations in serotonin levels in the brain may affect mood. Some antidepressant medications affect the action of serotonin, i.e. they are used to treat depression.

About 80% of our body's total serotonin is in the gut, in the enterochromaffin cells where it regulates intestinal movements. The rest is synthesized in the serotonergic neurons in the central nervous system.

For some types of cells, serotonin is a growth factor, it may have a role in wound healing.

Meditation increases the production of serotonin which is a calming neurotransmitter in the brain. The AIM Program incorporates activities and the Meditation CD which is an easy to use program to increase the levels of serotonin and other positive Control Points and thus improve general health.

Melatonin

Melatonin is a hormone produced by the pineal gland and helps to create restful sleep. The inability to sleep soundly can dramatically decrease the quality of your life and greatly speed up the aging process. The production of this important hormone rapidly declines with age. New research also reveals that Melatonin is a powerful antioxidant. In truth, it even more powerful than Vitamin E. Meditation increases the levels of melatonin in the body. Improving the natural production of melatonin is included in the AIM Program.

"By quieting the mind, which then quiets the body, and the less turbulent the body is, the more the self-repair healing mechanisms get amplified. In fact, scientists have shown that the better your DNA, your genetic machinery is at healing itself, the longer you live. That's how meditation lowers biological age." Deepak Chopra

Insulin

Insulin is the final hormone in the list of Control Points included in the AIM Program.

Insulin is a hormone that is important for metabolism and utilization of energy from the ingested nutrients, especially glucose.

Insulin is a protein chain or peptide hormone. There are 51 amino acids in an insulin molecule.

Insulin is produced in the islets of Langerhans in the pancreas. The name insulin comes from the Latin "insula" for "island" from the cells that produce the hormone in the pancreas.

Insulin has several broad actions including:

- It causes the cells in the liver, muscle, and fat tissue to take up glucose from blood and convert it to glycogen that can be stored in the liver and muscles
- Insulin also prevents the utilization of fat as an energy source. In absence of insulin or in conditions where insulin is low glucose is not taken up by body cells, and the body begins to use fat as an energy source.
- Insulin also controls other body systems and regulates the amino acid uptake by body cells
- It has several other anabolic effects throughout the body as well.
- Insulin is synthesized in significant quantities only in beta cells in the pancreas. It is secreted primarily in response to elevated blood concentrations of glucose. Insulin thus can regulate blood glucose and the body senses and responds to a rise in blood glucose by secreting insulin.

Other stimuli like sight and taste of food, nerve stimulation and increased blood concentrations of other fuel molecules, including amino acids and fatty acids, also promote insulin secretion.

- What happens when there is insufficient insulin?
- Since insulin controls the central metabolic processes, failure of insulin production leads to a condition called diabetes mellitus. There are two major types of diabetes – type 1 and type 2.
- Type 1 diabetes occurs when there is no or very low production of insulin from the pancreatic beta cells. Patients with Type 1 diabetes mellitus depend on external insulin (most commonly injected subcutaneously) for their survival.
- In type 2 diabetes mellitus the demands of insulin are not met by the amount produced by the pancreatic beta cells. This is termed insulin resistance or "relative" insulin deficiency. These patients may be treated with drugs to reduce their blood sugar or may eventually require externally supplied insulin if other medications fail to control blood glucose levels adequately.

When we eat, the body converts most substances to glucose (a type of sugar) and it flows through the blood. The cells use insulin to allow glucose to enter the cell to be used as fuel. When the cells are insulin resistant not enough glucose (fuel) enters the cells and glucose levels build up in the blood (high blood sugar) and cells are starved of the energy they need. When we have the condition over a longer period of time we began to exhibit a long list of health problems.

Many of the symptoms of diabetes can be overcome or minimized to the extent that medicines can be reduced with your doctor's guidance. When I first started developing the AIM Program I was not in contact with my doctor often enough and as a consequence I was taking too much medicine for my improving condition. The result was that I lost my driver's license for six months while I worked at convincing the DMV I have good enough control of my blood sugar to regain my license.

You will find hard copy journals included as a part of the AIM Program to keep you aware of your health condition and to keep your doctor informed. It is important that your doctor know about your involvement in the AIM Program so they can adjust your medicines as you continue on this wonderful journey.

In Chapter Three we are going to take a look at the situations that bring about improvements in our health. In Chapter Four we will take a look at the tools that will be used in the AIM Program. Up to this point the Program has all been theory but we will begin to include the "doing" part of the program. We will begin to explore how the mechanisms of the body are affected by the activities we are undertaking. We will begin to understand how something as simple as self esteem affects our Control Point hormones and thus our weight and general health. Let's face it, weight is simply a reflection of our general health.

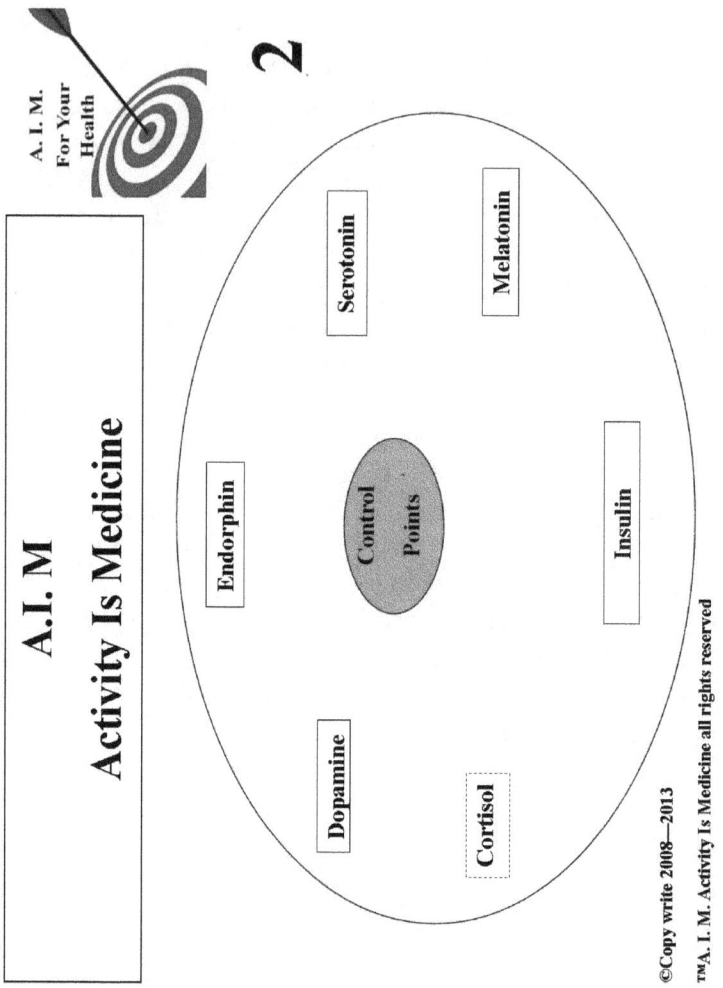

A.I. M
For Your
Health

A.I. M

Activity Is Medicine

Serotonin

Melatonin

Endorphin

Control Points

Insulin

Dopamine

Cortisol

2

The situations that bring about improved health

In Chapter One we discussed many of the situations that can cause poor health. In Chapter Two we looked at the Control Point Hormones that bring about improved health. As you saw, it is the increase of positive hormones (i.e. dopamine, endorphin and serotonin) and the reduction of negative hormones (i.e. Cortisol) that perform their magic in returning us to health. You can't go to your local pharmacy and get dopamine or endorphin. The good news is that your brain and other organs in your body will make the necessary hormones in the quantities you need if you take the actions to encourage production of those hormones.

For example: let's say your cortisol level is elevated causing you to feel nervous and upset and you want to reduce it. Take a walk for 45 minutes or an hour and cortisol levels will be reduced and also dopamine and endorphin levels will increase. You can also reduce cortisol and increase dopamine and endorphin by petting your cat, having sex, watching a sunset or meditating.

There are some very interesting facts involved here: One; you did not have to take a pill or inject a substance to get the results; two; you had to take some action (physical or mental) which puts the improvement of you health squarely in your hands; and three; the activities are low cost, easy to do and can be done on your schedule.

You will see the graphic at the end of this chapter includes other activities such as fellowship, positive feedback, improved self-esteem, re-engagement and of course proper nutrition all contributing to your improved health.

Let's take a look at one of my favorite situation that causes us poor health. At first it sounds so silly but as you look at it in relation to positive and negative hormone it makes so much sense. The situation I am talking about is positive or negative feedback. We start out life as a young child that is learning so rapidly all of the life skills necessary. We learn to sit up, walk, tie our shoes, use the potty, as well as get along with others. Then we go to school and the learning continues. With each lesson learned, with each task accomplished we are getting positive feedback that is building positive hormone levels.

If you are one of the people that have retired, so much of what you relied on for feedback is gone. No more new information to learn, no more schedules to meet and you have reduced interaction with other workers. Is it any wonder that when we retire our health starts going downhill? We really have to structure our lives to include mental and physical challenges.

In the next chapter (four) we will be starting the "doing" part of the AIM Program. The forth chapter begins to build the structure to encourage the production of the positive hormones

In Chapter Two we discussed serotonin and explained that about 80% of this great hormone is produced in the gut. Think back to a time when you were constipated or scared. You feel lethargic, get a belly ache, unable to think clearly and even get skin eruptions as the body's response to our food not passing quickly through our nutrient extraction equipment. We call this equipment the gut and it is made up of a number of sections where various processes take place.

This is a good place to point out the fact that food never directly enters the body. You never see a piece of steak floating in your blood. The easiest way to think about the gut or nutrient extraction equipment is to visualize a very long tube (about 30 feet) that starts at the mouth and ends at the anus. It is almost like a recycling disassembly moving beltline where the food is processed and various work stations remove the nutrients they need and pass the food on to the next work station. You can see that if we are getting enough fiber it gives the process greater bulk and makes the mass easier to process along the line. When we are not getting enough fiber the process slows down and enzymes began their natural food break down process into a rotting, smelly, gas producing mess. When our food turns toxic the liver gets involved and processes the toxin into fat and lipoids. Is it any wonder we get fat and our cholesterol increases when we don't get proper nutrition, which includes good amounts of fiber? We have been told over and over again we need good amounts of fiber and now we know why.

Let's talk for a minute about medicine, both prescribed and over the counter. Medicines are designed to reduce a specific symptom. They are foreign substances and appear to the body as a toxin. The liver sets about getting rid of them and flushing them from our body before they cause real damage.

Often times that process breaks down, for any number of reasons, and the toxic effects of the very medicine we are taking to reduce a symptom causes a whole new set of problems. We call them side effects and many times the side effects are worse than the problem we are trying to correct. Let me repeat: medicines are toxins. If you don't believe that statement, just read the vast list of side effects printed on all that cautionary paper work that comes with your prescription.

The goal should be to reduce the amount of medicines necessary to keep you functioning. You may never get off all medicine but you can reduce the amounts using the natural healing methods used throughout the AIM Program. My definition of natural healing includes exercise, nutrition and meditation. Those are the conventional methods that even the conventionally trained health care professional all seem to agree on. The AIM Program, however, goes a number of steps further. Rather than calling them therapy we refer to them as life styles. In therapy we tend to go somewhere or do some activity and then when we improve we stop and go back to our style of life. With the AIM Program we ask you to make a change in your style of life that includes small changes that will serve you throughout your life.

Some of the natural healing methods will include journalizing your health indicators everyday as a part of your routine just like brushing your teeth. Science has found that the simple act of recording your health measurements encourages the body to improve. Let's face it; the only cure comes from the body returning to full vibrant and joyous health. Affirmation also encourage the body to produce positive hormone and decrease cortisol.

Other natural healing methods will include repeating affirmations. Saying "we are enjoying good health" encourages the brain to go about its days looking for all of the things that will bring about good health.

We will also ask you to get into brain challenges to work that facility just like we work our muscles. We will show you methods to include activity into your lifestyle and remember, "Activity Is Medicine". We will show you how to include positive feedback, how to decrease your stress, increase fellowship, improve your self-esteem, re-engage with society and develop a positive outlook. I know, these may not sound like "natural healing methods" that we have been told all our lives. Once you begin to understand the mechanisms involved in encouraging the body's production of the "Control Point" hormones you will understand how thoughts and actions bring about health or disease. I will say it again "your health is in your hands".

Isn't it funny that our highly trained and highly paid health care professionals are not telling you that? The main reason they are not trained in it and they can't see a way to make money at it. It is starting to change. I heard a doctor on the Doctor Oz show say that to improve your health you should reduce stress by getting out of that toxic relationship, meditate, pay attention to getting more exercise and improve you intake of fresh fruits and vegetables. Wow! He is one of the first doctors I have heard that got it right.

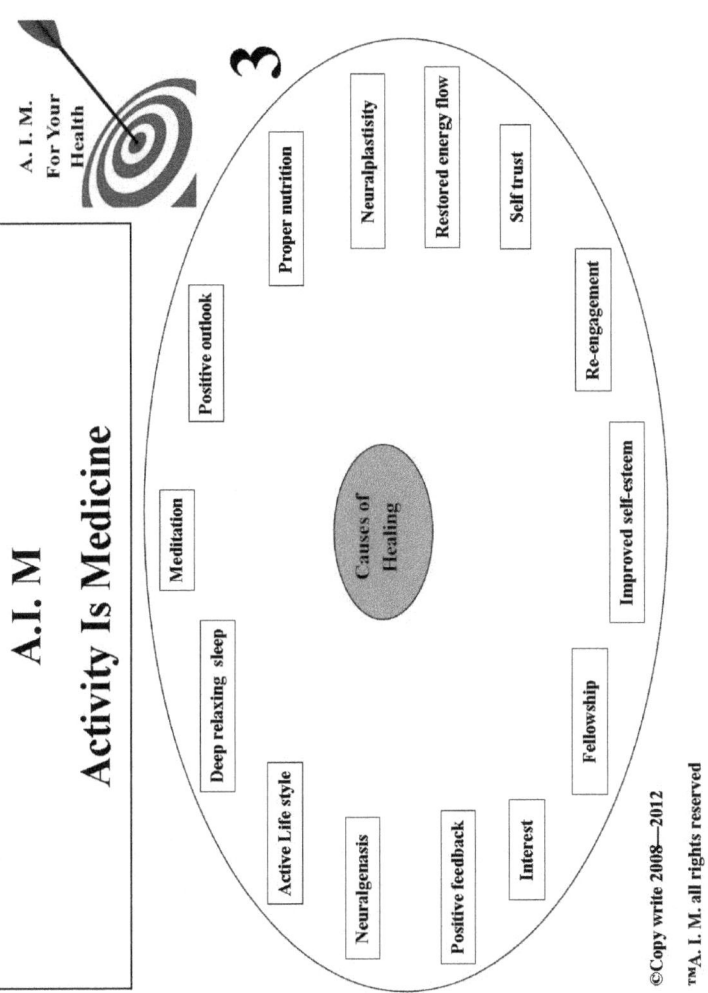

A. I. M
Activity Is Medicine

A. I. M.
For Your
Health

Causes of Healing

Proper nutrition
Neuralplastisity
Restored energy flow
Self trust
Positive outlook
Re-engagement
Meditation
Improved self-esteem
Deep relaxing sleep
Fellowship
Active Life style
Neuralgenasis
Positive feedback
Interest

Getting started with the AIM Program

Up to this point we have discussed why we lose our health, gain weight, and have trouble being as mentally sharp as we once were. We can blame it all on age but the truth is it has more to do with being inactive in so many ways and carrying around more negative thoughts. Our body is busy rebuilding every second of our lives. Yes, there is some slow down because of age but, there is so much we can do to help build our body and minds if we make it a greater priority.

The worse social invention we have developed is the concept of retirement. We get it into our head that once we reach a certain age we should slow down. We think that we should just lean back and take life easy. The fact is that as we age, people lose muscle mass and strength, flexibility and bone. The biggest cause is the lack of use, not aging. It is also a fact that through exercise we can gain muscle mass, strength, flexibility and bone. The statement "use it or lose it" is really true and pertains to both physical and mental health.

There is no evidence that the human body was built to function in a relaxed state. In fact, there is a large body of scientific evidence pointing to lack of activity as one of the most egregious cause of our modern health problems. The list of the health conditions that inactivity has been implicated in, reads like a handbook of what is wrong with the modern human. Some of the health issues implicated in inactivity are: risk of stroke, risk of heart attack, diabetes, joint pain, high blood pressure, reduced cognitive function, obesity and on, and on.

An active life style has been shown to reduce the risk of stroke, reduce the risk of heart attack, lower the effects of diabetes, reduce joint pain, lower blood pressure and improve cognitive function and reduce the incidence of obesity.

Here is just one side effect of exercise that can make a big change in your body's ability to heal itself. "Exercise helps the body make an enzyme that reduces the fat in your blood stream". How great is that?

This would be a good place to explain my perception of what is included in the definition of activity.

As you will remember in Chapter One we looked at what causes our health problems and we saw that one of the identified causes is inactivity. We have shown that there is not just one cause. So when we talk about inactivity, we can't equate inactivity with the lack of exercise only. Inactivity includes not exercising our brain, not engaging with society, not having mental harmany and therefore not getting good feedback.

My definition of activity includes an entire lifestyle of stretching the mind and challenging the body. It doesn't hurt and it becomes so much fun and you feel so good that you sometimes wonder if something is wrong with you that you feel that good.

The lack of activity leads to frailty which then leads to a loss of mobility and independence. Here is a quote from *PERSONAL HEALTH by JANE E. BRODY*. "This fact may sound discouraging. But it can be countered by another. Regular participation in aerobics, strength training and balance and flexibility exercises can delay and may even prevent a life-limiting loss of physical abilities into one's 90s and beyond".

Exercise doesn't mean you have to join a gym, hire a personal trainer or run a marathon to get the amount of exercise you need to get the kind of benefits you need to change your life. Walking is one of the best ways to get exercise and I never broke a sweat in my return to health. Just so you know I have lost forty pounds, ten inches around my belly, and my doctor has taken me off most of my medicine. The greatest benefit has been getting off medicine. You will find out later that medicine is actually a foreign substance and is handled by the liver as a toxin. The liver can make fat out of it and lipoids (bad cholesterol). Trying to fix something with medicine is like covering up the symptoms but never brings about a cure.

Being able to reduce the amount of medicine is one of the best benefits of the AIM program. The body will always pay a price for consuming medicines, which usually have toxic effects. The "side effects" are not the only toxic effect of medications. Doctors learn in their introductory pharmacology course in medical school that all medications are toxic to varying degrees, whether side effects are experienced or not. Pharmacology professors stress never to forget that. You cannot escape the immutable biological laws of cause and effect through ingesting medical substances. Taking drugs prescribed by physicians will not improve our health or extend our lives. Most prescribed drugs are not cures but reduce the symptoms and as soon as you stop using them the symptoms return. Fuhrman, Joel (2011-01-05). *Eat to Live: The Amazing Nutrient-Rich Program for Fast and Sustained Weight Loss (p. 25). Little, Brown and Compastony.* Kindle Edition.

So, there you have it. The AIM Program is not a diet; it is not an exercise program but a program that includes both, in addition to other components that address all of those divergent reasons that causes poor health.

Most of our members start the AIM Program within the Walking part of the system and gradually get into meditation, brain building, and improved nutrition. The program looks different to different people because they may find a part of the program that resonates with them and that may not be the same thing that resonates with their friends.

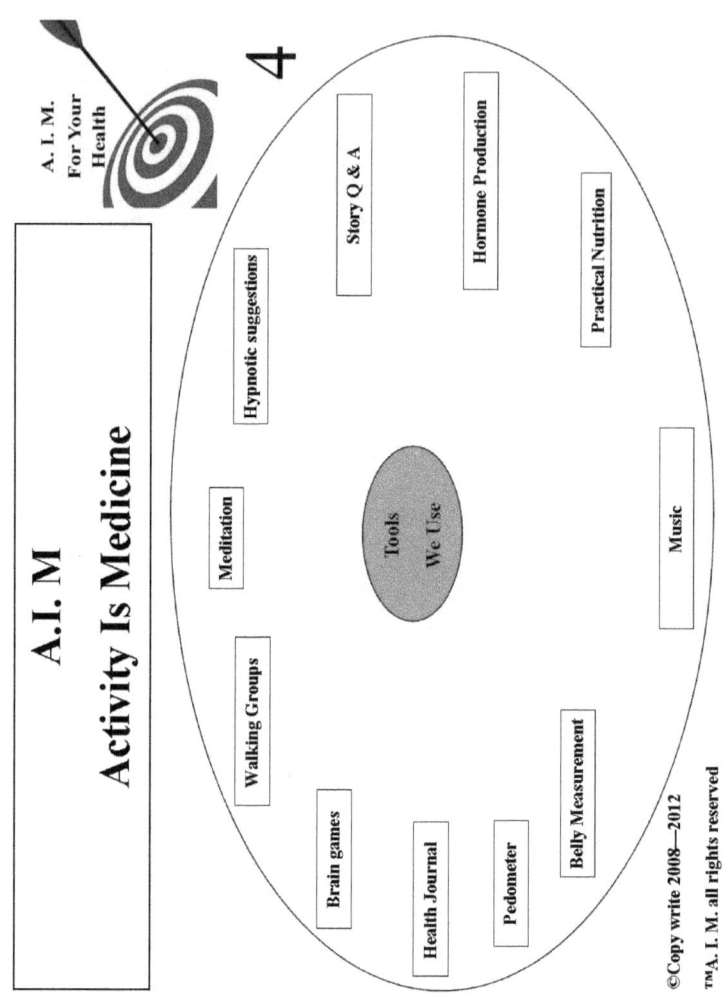

Time to get started

Getting started is easy and you can add components gradually as your health begins to improve.

Walking: The simple act of walking is one of the best ways to add activity to your life style. Many people don't think they can walk because of a bad hip or a bad knee. If you will start with just a few minutes a day and gradually increase the time you walk you will be surprised how the body will heal the problem. As with any new physical program, we suggest you ask your doctor if you are healthy enough to start walking.

The best walking programs are when you walk with a friend. Ask them to join you and you may be surprised to find out how many people want to get started but keep putting it off. Ask your neighbors, if you are like most people you don't know anyone further than a few houses away but this could be a good excuse to get to know what might turn out to be some very nice people.

Make sure you get everyone's phone number if they indicate an interest in joining your walking group. Call a small meeting to make some plans.

Starting or Joining an A. I. M. Walking Group

Find other people who are interested in walking

Go to the web site/bloog and search for people in your area and make contact.

Survey at least one preferred walking route with no dogs, broken sidewalks, or too steep hills.

Decide what day and time you want to get started.

Walk for a few days to see if you enjoy each others company

Go to the website and order "The Tool"

When you have all received your Tool Kits have a small "Kick Off Meeting".

Have someone bring a measuring tape, and a weight scale and be sure to have one or more blood pressure meters available.

Start by filling out your Walking Groups Buddy card so you all have each other's names and phone numbers.

Complete the General Health Journal

- Line one is the Bio-Metric Base Line reading that will be used to measure progress.
- Take and record the blood pressure (take three or four reading and record the lowest).
- Record the heart rate (the machine will record the pulse along with the pressure so use the lowest number.
- Take and record your blood sugar (even if not diabetic) because it is a good general health indicators.
- Measure the belly size at the core at the belly button (suck it in), we want to measure fat not weak muscles.
- Record the weight and height.
- Calculate the BMI (Body Mass Index from the chart) and record.
- Every, day - the blood pressure, pulse, blood sugar, steps taken (from the pedometer) should be taken and recorded. The other numbers should be taken every 3 to 4 weeks.

Setting Goals

- Your goals are to be recorded on the Goals Journal. Most start by setting a goal of getting into skinny jeans two sizes smaller then they currently have. It is so much fun to set goals and then gradually reach them. Also, don't forget to reward yourself.
- Start by setting short range goals (two months or less).
- Goals have to be measurable such as: lose 20 pounds or reduce blood pressure by 10 points.
- Goals must also have a time line such as: by January 2013, or by the end of the second quarter of 2014.
- Goals should be reachable but yet stretching.
- An example of a good goal might be: I chose to lose two dress/pant sizes by (date. Another worthwhile goal might be: I chose to work on the AIM Program and keep in touch with my doctor until I can get off of the high blood pressure medicine.
- Your next goal should be to get into your skinny jeans which are two sizes smaller than you currently wear.
- The plan is to have a party where all of the group can wear their skinny jeans or your take a day trip and all wear their skinny jeans. All have to wear the skinny jeans since it encourages the group to work together.

- You can get your skinny jeans from the back of your closet or buy used and place them where you can see them.
- Vary the walking route to add interest but be sure someone walks it first.
- Call each other at least every other day to keep the momentum going.
- Share your reading and take an interest in your partner's progress.
- When someone new enters the group, take them on as a mentor and help them out.
- Ask everyone you meet or know if they would be interested in joining a walking group.
- Have them join your group for a few times to get the feel of walking in a group.
- Have them go to the web site if they wish to walk with people closer to home and find someone closer (www.activityismedicine.com).
- Tell family and friends
- Mention your walking group to people in other areas. It doesn't really matter where they live since they can walk anywhere and maybe you can help them get started. It just feels go to help others.

The Daily Routine

The Daily Routine is important because it helps guide you through getting started correctly. It also keeps you headed in the right direction you have chosen.

Get Your Outlook Right

We know that our thoughts, attitudes and perceptions have a great effect on our health. It makes sense to adjust our outlook before we start the day.

Lay quietly before you jump out of bed and think of seven thinks you are thankful for. Eyes closed, relaxed and just think of seven things you are thankful for. Say thank you. Thank you. Thank you.

Giving Thanks

Giving thanks helps you and the "source" direct your thoughts and therefore your actions into a focused direction. There is some thought that giving thanks directs the source to give you more of the positive situations you are giving thanks for. Putting your mind in the thankfulness mode encourages the brain to produce more dopamine and keeps you in a positive mental outlook. Write it in your gratitude journal.

General Health Indicators

Taking and recording your general health indicators allows you to see your progress at the conscious as well as the subconscious level. As you progress, your mind gets excited about improving you progress. Your health improvement again encourages the brain to produce dopamine, endorphin, serotonin and melatonin all of which further improves your health.

Affirmations

Reading your affirmations out loud or to yourself in the mirror helps you adjust your attitude and perceptions into a more positive direction. You can use the supplied affirmation card to get started and later make you own version of an affirmation list customized to your life.

Writing Your Life's Direction

Writing your life plan helps the subconscious brain find the situations, people and events necessary to bring about the life you want. You start by making up the lifestyle you want in your mind and then putting it down on paper. You can get started by filling out the "Write Your New Life's Story" form you will find in your AIM Kit.

The Fat Flush Drink

You can start by using the included "Fat Flush" receipt included in the workbook. After using the receipt for a time I began to change it and look for other fruits and vegetables that I liked. Please feel free to change it around with one understanding. Our body's needs a wide variety of vitamins, minerals and fiber so changing the receipt can help you body get what it needs. Listen to your gut feel about how to change the receipt.

Here are some of the things I have found out about the receipt:

• Try to add some type of protein to each batch. I have used milk, a raw egg, peanut butter or a protein power. Be careful with protein power since most are made out of wheat so be sure you are not allegoric.

• Also include a probiotic such as yogurt. I have used regular yogurt and Greek yogurt and both work well.

• I try to add a hand full of nuts or seeds to boost the protein and the fiber of the finished drink. I found I have an allergy to raw peanuts but not peanut butter so I throw in a couple of spoons full of peanut butter.

• You can use water or milk for the fluid to mix it all up with. My personal favorite is to brew about 10 cups of green tea at night and put it in the refrigerator. In the morning I use some of the tea mix for the receipt. Again, you can use green tea, black tea, white tea or blossom teas in any combination.

• Each receipt I make includes three fruits and/or two to three vegetables and it is seldom the same from one day to the next,

The AIM Meditation CD

Listening to the AIM CD for just twenty minutes a day three to five days a week can make measurable changes in your outlook and health.

Stress and the side effects of stress cause the liver to make fat and store it in the midsection. And that is only one of the bad things about stress. Stress brings about increases in cortisol and cortisol starts killing cells after about 20 minutes. Although cortisol is very necessary in stressful situations but that quickly turns into a toxin which, long term, causes disease. Meditation and posthypnotic suggest can help reduce levels of cortisol and teach our subconscious mind how to better handle stress and quickly put stressful situations into better perceptions.

Stress and negative outlook also decreases levels of good hormones such as dopamine, endorphins, serotonins, and melatonin. Reductions in these good hormones can put you in a negative outlook, make it more difficult to accomplish things and not sleep well. This can cause a downward spiral that may take a change in life style to get back on track.

Often times we are ready to make meaningful changes in our life style but habits are so strong we find ourselves slipping back to our old habits in a short period of time. The AIM series of posthypnotic suggest CDs can be a big help in unconsciously changing your life style to live the life you want.

Science has shown that meditation can increase levels of positive hormones, decrease cortisol and change thought patterns to bring about positive changes in life style without conscious effort.

Listen to the AIM CD and give it a few days. You will find your outlook more positive and you will find your general health indicators start to improve.

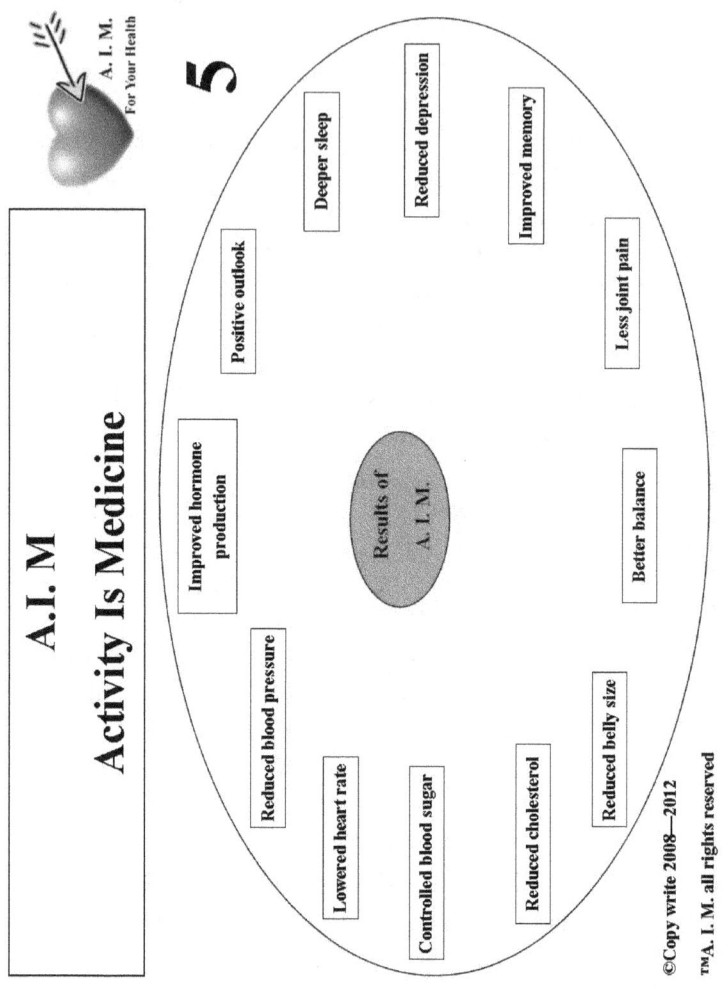

A. I. M.
For Your Health

A.I. M
Activity Is Medicine

Results of
A. I. M.

Improved hormone production

Positive outlook

Deeper sleep

Reduced depression

Improved memory

Less joint pain

Better balance

Reduced blood pressure

Lowered heart rate

Controlled blood sugar

Reduced cholesterol

Reduced belly size

©Copy write 2008—2012

™A. I. M. all rights reserved

Re-engaging in life

It is an interesting phenomenon that when we retire and children have moved on, we tend to disconnect from our family, long term friends and general society. We lose our life's structure and have to make up our new life style. When do we get up? When do we go to bed? What do we spend our time doing with our new freedom during the day? We start watching TV more, spending less time struggling to learn new information, and we settle into a more relaxed style of life.

If you are newly retired or have been retired for some time you will begin to see children moving on with their own life and the invitations to special events become further and further apart if at all. I have seen it in my own life. Children go to school, get jobs, move out, come back once or twice, and they have children of their own. Then comes their own involvement with their children's schools, sports teams, and general life activities and grand mom and dad are left to lead their own disconnected life.

Now, you, the grandparents are left to your own devices. Before you know it you find it is so much easier to sit around and watch TV than make your own entertainment. Because you are not challenging your brain and body the way you were use to in your younger years. Your health begins to deteriorate and the poor health "downward spiral" begins.

This is exactly where the AIM Program kicks in to help you change your lifestyle. Now this is your time of your life. You still can do or become anything you want but, first we have to get your health back on track.

Remember, there are a number of reasons that we get sick, fat and have a brain fog. Being with others challenges our brain and increases our good hormones and that makes us stronger mentally and physically.

When we take a class, go to a work out course or write an article, attend a seminar, call our grandkids, or an old friend we have not talked to in years, we involve our brain in new ways. We can enroll in a class in a new subject or an advanced class in a subject we love which again increase the challenges to our brain.

It is not just exercise, it is not just nutrition, it is not just positive feedback...it is all of it and more. Who has ever told you this? You have known it deep in your gut that it takes a whole lot of changes in your life style to bring you back to great health. Once you have your great health back you can move on to all of those things you want to accomplish in your "second act".

Once I got my health back I went back to work. This time I am a maintenance man at the hotel right next to the apartment building I live in. Talk about a short commute! The real message here is that once you get your great health back you can't just sit around and watch TV all day. You have so much energy you have to get involved with life. Working an eight hour day five days a week does not leave much time to some things but you does learn to balance it and move ahead.

What do we do to get back into a life style that challenges us and makes us a more interesting person to be around? Start small; join a class at your local senior center. Remember, back in the day, when you wanted to become a ....you fill in the blank. Getting your health back opens up a life of more energy and you start believing you really can do, become, or have that which you have been dreaming of most of your life.

The AIM Program is designed to get you started and keep you going on the patch to a better, more rewarding life.

Let's get started with the daily routine. We need routines to help guide that wild bucking bronco we call our mind. Left to its self it will run off in a thousand different directions. The daily routine helps you establish habits that are both health giving and good patterns of life.

Following the daily routine, will first off, get you to look at and record you daily general health indicators. With just a little activity and the positive feedback of your general health indicators and things will begin to happen and for the better.

One of the first ways to get reconnected with society and your family and friends is to stop watching so much TV.

Researchers have shown that watching TV causes your brain waves to slow down from beta to alpha. For example, psychophysiology Thomas Mulholland decided to measure the attention spans of children. He programmed an EEG machine which measures brain waves, to turn off the TV set whenever the kids produced more alpha than beta waves. Then he challenged the kids to concentrate as hard as they could in order to keep the TV on. Much to his amazement, most of the kids couldn't keep the TV set on for more than half a minute. That's how little time it takes to lull our brains into that hypnotic state. From: *Harmonic Wealth by James Arthur Ray.*

The second change you need to make in your life style is to change your belief system. "What you believe you'll achieve": This statement is the driving factor of your results for your lack of abundance in terms of money, peace of mind, relationships, physical health, or anything else. The AIM Program addresses this statement and puts it into practical application with: 1. Affirmations, 2. Setting your goals, 3. Starting a Walking Group, 4. Writing your new life's story, 5. Meditation CD's, and 6. Posthypnotic suggestions CD's. "Change the film you play over and over in your mind and you change your results".

The world is calling for you to master your mind and change your attitude and your beliefs and become what you hold dear. The world needs you to be fully engaged again and sharing with us the fully expressed extraordinary you.

Brain Games

We all start noticing a decrease in our mental skills as we age. Neuroscientists now say that there is no physical reason that we should lose brain power. They have tracked it down to a lack of challenging our brain to continue to make new neurons, synapse and brain fluid. The neurons are the place where we store our memory and have multiply connections to other neurons. Those connections are called dendrites and are the physical wiring connections to other neurons. Neurons can have connections to hundreds of other neurons to makeup the complexity of our thinking, reasoning and decision making.

It is common knowledge that we "use it or lose it" and that pertains to our brain as well as our body. Science has shown that mental exercises "of all different types" rebuilds brain parts in a process called neurogenesis.

Take care of your physical brain through nutrition to insure a healthy brain function. The AIM Program will lead you through the "practical nutrition" to bring about improved health. Did you know the brain only weighs 2% of our total body weight yet it consumes over 20% of the total oxygen and nutrients we intake? To supply this enormous requirement of vitamins, minerals and oxygen we need lots of good nutritious food to feed our brain as well as our physical and mental needs. In addition, the brains function and very structure needs omega-3 fatty acids and that only comes from our diet and supplements.

The brain is so complex and keeping it challenged requires a wide array of tools worked on every day. The tools include brain games, brain puzzles, and changes in all aspects of your life as well as others.

Brain challenges do not need to be hard or complicated but they do need to be consistence. This is why AIM introduces Brain Games and the latest scientific research by our weekly e-mail newsletter. To take full advantage of the life healing benefits of the AIM Program is sure we have your e-mail address so you can start getting your weekly newsletter. If you are not getting your news letter, please go to our web site at: www.activityismedicine.com/bloog and sign up. The first three months are free and come with your starter kit.

Practical nutrition

Practical Nutrition is the process of eating a diet that makes practical sense no matter what your ethnic background may be.

I tried all of the diets hopping to lose weight but all that ever happened was I spent meals choking down terrible tasting food. After I could not take it any longer I gave up on that diet and moved back to my ethnic engrained eating patterns and gained more weight.

I tried various diets feeling that if I could lose weight I might get my health back. The problem is I could lose weight but it did not seem to change my overall health. After months and months of reviewing scientific research I found that what we need to do is to get our health back and the body will adjust its natural weight. So excess weight is a good indicator of general health and when you get your health back the body sheds the weight. WOW! What a concept. Gain your health and lose the weight. I think we tend to focus on losing weight and our health gets even worse.

So here is the thing. Don't worry about the weight. In the AIM Program we try not to weigh ourselves for the first four months. We concentrate on measuring inches around our belly and our general health indicators and the weight will take care of itself.

Let's get back to Practical Nutrition. I found out by reading books by nutritionists, medical doctors and libratory research papers that what the body needs is nutrients of all types. Scientists call them macro and micro nutrients.

There are three primary macronutrients defined as being the classes of chemical compounds humans consume in the largest quantities and which provide bulk energy. These are protein, fat, and carbohydrate. Macronutrients can also refer to the chemical elements humans consume in the largest quantities. Micronutrients are nutrients humans require in small quantities throughout life. These are micronutrients: macro minerals, organic acids, trace minerals and vitamins. If we don't get sufficient quantities of each of the macro and micro nutrients our health will suffer.

The AIM Program typically starts members in the Practical Nutrition portion of the program in a number of ways.

We suggest that you eat what you have always eaten but just a little less. Reduce your food intake by about 10% to 20%. We don't want to introduce too many changes in your life style too fast as you will find yourself back at square one.

Stand in front of your mirror and read your affirmations. Your subconscious mind has got to believe you are getting healthy before it can happen. Read your affirmations 3 to 5 days a week.

Introduce some sort of activity and we recommend walking to get started. The increase of calories burned with the addition of reduced calories input will start the process in the right direction.

Listen to the AIM Program CD at least five out of seven days.

Make you morning Micronutrient shake and enjoy it five out of seven days. I usually make enough for two days at once, and put half in the refrigerator, so I only need to make a new batch every third day.

Later in the program, in our weekly news letter, we will take up the question of the best ways to get the micro and macro nutrients. You will also learn practical suggestions for how to read the nutritional label and most importantly, the ingredients. What foods to chose and more.

The value of walking

How good is walking...really

Did you know that every minute you walk can extend your life by 1.5 to 2 minutes? In addition, many studies show that people, who walk regularly live longer, weigh less, have lower blood pressure, and enjoy better overall health than non-walkers.

Are you ready to lace on your shoes? If you want to add to the amount of walking you do, just clip on a pedometer. That simple action actually increases your physical activity by over 2100 steps per day, a review that pooled data from 26 studies found.

Here's a look at ten benefits of walking.

Walking Increases Your Lifespan

Walking more than an hour a day improves life expectancy significantly, a 2011 study showed. The researchers looked at 27,738 participants between the ages of 40 and 79 over a 13-year period. Surprisingly, their lifetime medical costs did not increase—even though they lived longer.

"An increase in walking time at the population level would bring about a tremendous change in people's health and medical cost," the study authors wrote.

Walking Wards off Diabetes

Just thirty minutes of walking a day can prevent diseases such as type 2 diabetes. A 2002 study looking at both overweight and average weight men and women in a population at high risk for the disease showed a reduction in risk factors.

If you already have diabetes, walking is helpful for you, too. A mile or more daily cuts your risk of death from all causes in half, according to a 2007 study.

Walking Keeps Your Mind Sharp

Walking 72 blocks a week (around six to nine miles) helps increase grey matter, which in turn lowers the risk of suffering from cognitive impairment—or trouble with concentration, memory and thought, according to a study which looked at 299 seniors over a nine-year period.

Furthermore, walking five miles per week can provide some protection to the memory and learning areas of the brains of those already suffering from Alzheimer's disease or mild cognitive impairment, and lead to a slower decline in memory loss.

Walking Helps Lower Blood Pressure
Walking just 30 minutes a day, three to five days a week—even when the 30 minutes are broken into three ten-minute increments—has been found to significantly lower blood pressure.

Walking is great for Bone Health
Putting one foot in front of the other for about a mile a day led to improved bone density in post-menopausal women, and slowed the rate of bone loss from the legs, according to a 1994 study. "It takes walkers four to seven years longer to reach the point of very low bone density, study leader Dr. Krall told the New York Times.

Walking Cuts the Risk of Stroke
Walking about 12.5 miles a week or more cut the risk of stroke in half, according to a study looking at over 11,000 Harvard University alumni with an average age of 58.

Walking Improves Your Mood
If you're feeling down in the dumps, walking is a quick and easy solution. Just thirty minutes on a treadmill reduces feelings of tension and depression, according to research published in the British Journal of Sports Medicine. In fact, the study found that walking lifted moods more quickly than anti-depressants did (and with fewer side effects).

And the more people walk, the better their mood and energy, says California State University Long Beach professor Robert Thayer, based on a study looking at 37 study participants over a 20-day period.

Walking Torches Calories
Just 20 minutes of walking a day will burn 7 pounds a year. The effects are even more dramatic when you add in some dietary changes as well.

Walking Improves Insomnia

Having trouble sleeping at night? Try taking a brisk 45-minute walk in the morning five days a week, and your sleep may improve significantly, according to research from the Fred Hutchinson Cancer Research Center in Seattle, which looked at women from the age of 50-74. (Walking in the evening, however, sometimes has the opposite effect—so keep an eye on when you're exercising and what your sleep patterns are.)

Walking is good for the Heart

Women who took brisk walks for three or more hours per week reduced their risk of heart disease by 30-40 percent, according to an analysis of over 72,000 women aged 40-65, who were enrolled in the prospective Nurses' Health Study. As I reported recently, heart attacks kill more US women than men annually. However, the benefits of walking aren't limited to one gender. A different study showed that walking can cut the risk of coronary heart disease in half for men between the ages of 71 and 93.

Here is A Summary

According to an article in "First for women" magazine 4/16/2012:

Walking Perks

10% better focus

50% sounder sleep

88% sunnier moods

90% improved confidence

20% less anxiety

29% fewer cravings

37% fewer aches and pains and 50% fewer sick days

Meditation

The A. I. M. Meditation CD

The AIM Meditation CD program guides the brain through various levels of brain wave frequencies. In certain brain wave frequencies the brain releases numerous highly beneficial substances, including (HGH) human growth hormone.

It is within delta that our brains are triggered to release great quantities of healing hormones, one of which is human growth hormone (HGH) which we make less of as we age, resulting in many symptoms and diseases associated with aging.

Hollywood stars pay up to $20,000 a year for synthetic human growth hormone injections, because it brings back youthful energy, looks, and stamina. The professional athletic organizations are working on outlawing it since it gives the athletics a great advantage. And I agree, the effects of HGH are dramatic: Greater muscle tone, stronger bones and less fat,

Increased brain function and younger-looking, tighter skin!

HGH is one of the reasons kids have endless energy—their pituitary glands spew out heaps of the stuff!

Unfortunately, your body produces less HGH as you get older—as much as 50% less by our late 50s.

And it shows!

But HGH injections are dangerous, expensive and can cause frightening side effects!!

Now you know you can produce HGH and many other healing hormones, naturally and safely with a little daily AIM meditation.

"By quieting the mind, which then quiets the body, and the less turbulent the body is, the more the self-repair healing mechanisms get amplified. In fact, scientists have shown that the better your DNA, your genetic machinery is at healing itself, the longer you live. That's how meditation lowers biological age. *Deepak Chopra*

As we become older, the brain creates lesser quantities of these beneficial substances and we therefore develop various ageing symptoms and diseases.

Recent research performed by Dr. Vincent Giampapa, M.D., a prominent anti-aging researcher and past-president of the American Board of Anti-Aging Medicine, revealed that regular deep meditation dramatically affects production of three important hormones related to increased longevity, stress, and enhanced well-being: cortisol, DHEA, and melatonin.

At the slower Alpha and Theta brainwave patterns, production of DHEA and melatonin increases significantly.

One study noted an increase in DHEA of as much as 44%. Some even had DHEA increases of up to 90%.

Melatonin increases were even more astounding, with average increases of 98% recorded. Many participants even had increases of up to 300%. Melatonin is a hormone produced by the pineal gland and helps to create restful sleep. The inability to sleep soundly can dramatically decrease the quality of your life and greatly speed up the aging process. The production of this important hormone rapidly declines with age.

New research also reveals that Melatonin is a powerful antioxidant. In truth, it is yet more powerful than Vitamin E. Meditation increases the levels of melatonin in the body.

On the other hand, cortisol levels declined by an average of 47%. Of course, not all study participants showed the same results, but about 70% of the study participants recorded the above improvements.

Cortisol is the major age-accelerating hormone

Cortisol is a hormone naturally produced by the adrenal glands. According to Dr. Giampapa, cortisol is the major age-accelerating hormone. It also interferes with learning and memory and is, in general, bad news for your health and your well-being.

Cortisol is the "stress hormone," and the more of it you have, the more stressed you feel...the more vulnerable to disease you are and the faster you age!

Now you know! You increase positive hormones and decrease negative hormones simply by listening to the Meditation CD's.

You can purchase them on our website at: www.activityismedicine.com.

We wish you the best of luck. Take it slow, these changes are making alterations in habits you have worked a lifetime to create. It is going to take some time to transform them. But, realize, it is not impossible, like learning to ride a bike.

Be sure to get someone else involved in your journey. Someone that will find the good in what you want to accomplish.

About the Author

Mr. Keiser, the author of this book and the developer of the A. I. M. Program is now 74 years old and has come from a fat, sick, and old man taking way to much medicine to a young 74 year old with lots of vitality, certainty and almost medicine free. He just wants lots of people to get their health back and wrote this book to bring that about. Let me allow him to tell you in his own words;

How the AIM Program Came About

When I look back at my life a few years ago I see an old man, sick with lots of medicines. I was a diabetic, with high blood pressure, lots of cholesterol, way overweight and a brain on the way out. I was like most of the people in my apartment building. I was spending most of my time being inactive, watching TV, reading and planning for my next doctor's visit so I could tell him how much my joints hurt. I really expected sympathy, but instead I got a lecture about the road I was heading down if I didn't change my life.

By this time I was about forty pounds overweight, with a belly that required a belt 10 inches longer than I needed when I had been a young man. My doctor said "Mr. Keiser, you are going to have to take this diabetes seriously or some bad things are going to start happening to you". He continued by saying "you are at very high risk of heart attack, stroke, sight loss and other bad things". When I asked him what I should do he said, "You are going to have to get active and lose weight". I asked him how I could do that. He really did not have the time to get into it but told me that my health care provider did some have some good classes that may help.

It wasn't until later when I started thinking about what it would be like once you had a stroke or heart attack if you lived through it. I hated the thought of being confined to a bed or wheel chair and having to have people take care of me. I loved the thought of living an independent life and going where I wanted to and when I wanted to. Although I was in my sixties I was just not ready to admit I was "old". I had seen plenty of seniors that continued an active and productive life and I wanted to be one of those people.

I signed up for the course on diabetes and looked forward to the day the class started. The class was a number of weeks in length and was held in a class room style. We got lots of information from people who were very well educated with lots of certificates. It was very apparent that these people did not have diabetes and were not going though what we were. We watched movies and slide presentations and carried home a major boat load of paper. I never heard from those people again. It was as if: here take this ton of information and figure out how to implement it in your life.

When I got home I tried to remember what the instructors said in class. I looked thought my written information to try to make sense of the life style changes I was going to have to make to turn things around. Wait... What? I was going to have to make changes in my life style? Oh, no I just want to take something to make it all better. That was where it really started. You find that all of that medicine does nothing to bring about a "cure". The next time you go to your doctor they increase the dosage or add an additional pill.

I wanted to find out what was causing my health problems and what would change it for the better. I didn't want to just take more and more medicine. I started reading everything I could find. I subscribed to newsletters from teaching hospitals, universities, laboratories, and governmental agencies, magazines and newspapers. My files started to fill up and my bank account when the other direction.

Often times I would find a pearl of wisdom that I could actually use in my life. The first real breakthrough was the discovery of the use of journalizing to record my health indicators on a daily basis. The indicators were ones we have all heard of. They were simple to do, could be done in my home without running to a lab every day. I could afford the equipment and they actually reflected what was going on. By writing things down I could see what was helping and what did not have much of an effect. Here is what I started recording every day, first time in the morning: blood pressure, heart rate, blood sugar, steps taken and my belly size. Notice I did not use weight since it is not a good reflection of general health. Journalizing was a real revelation on so many levels. I could see what made a difference and what didn't. I could begin to feel good about myself as things began to improve. I had real numbers to talk about not just subjective feelings. Now I could separate the "nice to know" information coming out of science from the information that had a practical application in my life and is effect.

The next direction my research had taken was to find out what causes poor health. By this time I had changed my career from a fat old retired guy to a health researcher.

Along the way I began to see that much of the scientific research being done is so narrow and specialized that it is hard to apply to our everyday life. But, never the less, I did find situations or things that have a negative effect on our health. Many things by themselves may have little effect but when a host of situations come together they can be really bad. Many of the things having a bad effect on our health are not the things health care professionals are warning us about. Here is a good example: loss of sleep, poor self concept, worry and disengagement with society. Many health care professionals tell us we need to be more active and get better nutrition.

I found that it is not that simple. Turns out that poor health is a complex of causes many of which we have never heard of but most of them are easy to change.

The first step is to look at what makes us sick, fat and old. The second step is to look at the control points that profoundly affect our health and our enjoyment in life and our very relationships with others. Step three is to look at what changes we can make in our style of life to bring about great and good health. Step four looks at what tools are included in the AIM Program to help you make the changes that will benefit your short term and long term health. The fifth chapter identifies the positive and delicious changes that have been proven by scientific research, personal experience and feedback from others involved in the AIM Program.

Be sure to get your "Starter Kit" from our website at: www.activityismedicine.com to get you started on this wonderful journey. Good luck and be sure to bring someone else along.

www.ingramcontent.com/pod-product-compliance
Lightning Source LLC
Chambersburg PA
CBHW070625290526
45790CB00002B/995